QUICK REFERENCE TO ABDOMINAL ULTRASONOGRAPHY

SANDRA L. HAGEN-ANSERT
BA, RDMS, RDCS

Program Director of Diagnostic Ultrasound,
Department of Radiology; formerly Clinical and Research
Echocardiographic Sonographer,
Pediatric Cardiology Division; Clinical Neonatal
Echoencephalographic Sonographer,
Neonatal Support Center, University of California,
San Diego Medical Center,
San Diego, California

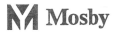

Mosby

ST LOUIS · BALTIMORE · BOSTON · CHICAGO · LONDON
MADRID · PHILADELPHIA · SYDNEY · TORONTO

Editor: Jeanne Rowland
Developmental Editor: Lisa Potts

FIRST EDITION
Copyright © 1995 by Mosby–Year Book, Inc.

Printed in the United States of America

Mosby–Year Book, Inc.
11830 Westline Industrial Drive
St. Louis, Missouri 63146

International Standard Book Number 0-8016-7949-4

94 95 96 97 98   /   9 8 7 6 5 4 3 2 1

PREFACE

This quick reference has been designed to provide easy access to information on abdominal sonography. It specifically covers the vascular and biliary system, the pancreas, the liver, the gallbladder, and the kidney, and abscess formation and pockets in the abdomen and pelvis.

Terminology is defined, and numerous pathologic conditions are described, including explanations of laboratory results, symptoms, sonographic findings, and causes. *Quick Reference to Abdominal Ultrasonography* presents information in a concise outline format so facts can be found within seconds.

Sandra L. Hagen-Ansert

CONTENTS

GENERAL SONOGRAPHY TERMINOLOGY

ANECHOIC: No internal echoes, enhanced posterior through transmission (example: bladder, gallbladder)

ECHOGENIC: Very bright echoes within a structure; i.e., more echo-dense than the liver parenchyma (example: gallstones, calcifications)

HOMOGENEOUS: Even texture throughout (example: normal liver parenchyma, normal spleen, placenta, uterus)

HETEROGENEOUS: Uneven echo texture (example: kidney)

HYPOECHOIC: Low level echoes in comparison to normal texture; i.e., enlarged lymph nodes are hypoechoic, or less echogenic than the normal liver parenchyma

HYPERECHOIC: Increased echoes in comparison to normal texture; i.e., hemangioma of the liver may show a bright, echogenic texture when compared to the normal liver texture

ABDOMINAL REGIONS, CAVITIES, AND SPACES TERMINOLOGY

ABDOMINAL CAVITY (excluding the retroperitoneum and pelvis): Bounded superiorly by the diaphragm, anteriorly by the abdominal wall muscles, posteriorly by the vertebral column, ribs, and iliac fossa, and inferiorly by the pelvis.

PERITONEUM: Thin, translucent, serous membrane that lines the walls of abdominal cavity and covers abdominal viscera. Has two layers:
- Parietal: Lines walls of abdominal cavity.
- Visceral: Covers abdominal organs.

Between the two layers is the peritoneal cavity, which contains a small amount of lubricating serous fluid for free movement. In the male, this cavity is closed; in the female, a communication with the exterior exists through the fallopian tubes, uterus, and vagina.

PERITONEAL CAVITY: Divided into two parts (greater and lesser sac)

GREATER SAC: Largest of the two peritoneal sacs and extends across the abdomen from the diaphragm to the pelvis.

LESSER SAC: Lies posterior to the stomach; as a small diverticulum from the greater sac. It opens through a window called the epiploic foramen.

MESENTERY: Two-layered fold of peritoneum that attaches part of the intestine to the posterior abdominal wall, including the small intestine, transverse colon, and sigmoid colon.

GREATER OMENTUM: Two-layered fold of peritoneum that

attaches the stomach to another viscera. It is often referred to as an apron hanging between the small intestine and the anterior abdominal wall and is attached to the greater curvature of the stomach.

LESSER OMENTUM: Attaches the lesser curvature of the stomach to the under surface of the liver.

- The visceral peritoneum covers the anterior surface of the stomach, and the lesser curvature forms the anterior layer of the lesser omentum.
- Has a free border on the right where it folds around the common bile duct, hepatic artery, and portal vein. This free border forms the anterior margin of the opening of the lesser sac.
- Peritoneum forms the posterior layer of the lesser omentum to become continuous with the visceral layer of the peritoneum covering the posterior stomach wall.

GASTROSPLENIC OMENTUM: Attaches the stomach to the spleen. The peritoneum leaves the greater curvature of the stomach to form the gastrosplenic omentum.

PERITONEAL LIGAMENTS: Attach the less mobile solid viscera to the abdominal walls. The mesenteric omenta and the peritoneal ligaments allow the blood vessels, lymphatics, and nerves to reach the other viscera in the abdomen.

- *FALCIFORM LIGAMENT*: Attaches the liver to the abdominal wall and diaphragm.
- *MEDIAN UMBILICAL LIGAMENT*(Urachus): Passes from the apex of the bladder to the umbilicus.
- *LATERAL UMBILICAL LIGAMENT*: Obliterated umbilical arteries. Pass from the internal iliac artery to the umbilicus.
- *LIGAMENTUM TERES*: Obliterated umbilical fetal vein. Passes upward to enter the groove between the medial segment and the lateral segment of the left lobe of the liver.
- *LIENORENAL LIGAMENT*: Peritoneal layer from kidney to the hilum of the spleen.

- *GASTROSPLENIC LIGAMENT*: Passes from the hilus of the spleen to the greater curvature of the stomach.

DUODENUM AND SMALL INTESTINE: Most of the digestion and absorption of food takes place in the small intestine, which is divided into three parts: duodenum, jejunum, and ileum.

STOMACH: Lies under the ribs in the left upper abdomen, and extends from the left hypochondriac region into the epigastric and umbilical regions.

- Two openings: Cardiac and pyloric orifices.
- Two curvatures: Lesser and greater.
- Two surfaces: Anterior and posterior.
- Divided into fundus, body, pyloric antrum, and pylorus.

GENERAL FLUID COLLECTIONS*

Lab/Symptoms
- Swelling or bloating of affected area with or without pain
- Fever

Sonography of Fluid Collections
- Assume shape of available space around collection.
- Change position with patient position.
- May contain septa.
- Important to separate bowel (peristalsis) from fluid.

---

*See also Abscesses and Pockets in the Abdomen and Pelvis.

VASCULAR

NORMAL AORTIC GROWTH PATTERNS: 3 cm or less abdominal aorta; 2 cm or less iliac artery; 1 cm or less femoral artery.

Sonography of the Aorta
- Anechoic tubular vessel with medium echo reflections from the aortic walls.

AORTIC ANEURYSMS
- In patients with aneurysm measuring 3.0 to 5.9 cm, annual growth is .23 to .28 cm.
- Aneurysms over 6 cm followed yearly
  - 75% pts (1) year survival if <6 cm.
  - 50% pts (1) year survival if >6 cm.
  - 25% pts (1) year survival if >7 cm.
  - 75% risk fatal rupture if >7 cm.
  - 1% rupture if <5 cm.

Cause
- Most common is atherosclerotic changes in the arterial wall; less common due to mycotic or dissecting lesions.

Types
1. *SACCULAR:* Only small connection to the aorta, one aspect of the wall diseased.
2. *FUSIFORM:* Most common at level of bifurcation, decreased pulsations, bright echoes reflecting degree of thickening and calcification.

3. *BERRY ANEURYSM:* Small spherical aneurysm 1.0 to 1.5 cm.

4. *DISSECTION:* Tear in the tunica intima.

MARFAN'S SYNDROME: Cystic medial necrosis leading to weakening of the aortic lumen with huge, dilated aneurysmal formation.

AORTIC GRAFT

Lab/Symptoms

- Previous surgery to repair aortic aneurysm.

Sonography

- Shows distinct, clear, well-defined borders, with brighter reflections from the graft material than from the normal aortic wall.

Complications

- Hematoma.
- Infection.
- Degeneration of graft material.
- False aneurysm formation at site.

AORTIC DISSECTION

May tear at one of three primary sites: root of aorta, level of left subclavian artery, abdominal aorta at level of crus.

Lab/Symptoms

- Back pain.
- Hypotension.
- Chest pain.
- Shock.

Causes

- Cystic medial necrosis.
- Marfan's syndrome.

- Hypertension.
- Previous aortic aneurysm.

Sonography
- Flap of tear is seen along tunica intima with blood escaping into channel with or without frank aneurysm dilation.

RUPTURED AORTIC ANEURYSM

Lab/Symptoms
- Increased abdominal pain, shock, expanding abdominal mass.

Notes: Operative mortality for rupture is 40-60%

COMPLICATIONS OF ANEURYSMS
- When large, may compress other structures, i.e., common bile duct or renal arteries.
- A high thoracic aneurysm may present as chest mass.
- Mycotic aneurysm may produce septic symptoms.

DIFFERENTIAL DIAGNOSIS OF ABDOMINAL ANEURYSM
Retroperitoneal mass, parotic nodes (lymphoma).

OTHER ANEURYSMS
CELIAC ARTERY: Anterior branch of aorta.
SUPERIOR MESENTERIC ARTERY: May occur secondary to pancreatitis.
SPLENIC OR HEPATIC ARTERY: Caused by atherosclerosis, infective emboli, congenital factors, trauma.
- Seen in portal hypertension.
- Females of childbearing age.
- Many patients asymptomatic.

Differential Diagnosis

- Pancreatic cyst.
- Segmental dilation of the pancreatic duct.
- Lymphadenopathy.
- Gastric varices.

RENAL ARTERY: Uncommon.

Causes

- Atherosclerosis
- Trauma
- Pregnancy
- Congenital anomaly
- Pelvic surgery
- Syphilis
- Bacterial infection

Notes

- 50% of aneurysms rupture if untreated.
- Most are extensions of abdominal aneurysm.
- May be isolated, usually bilateral.
- Measure from 3 to 8 cm.
- More common in men.

ARTERIOVENOUS FISTULAS

Majority are secondary to trauma (acquired).

Renal

- Congenital: Crisoid or aneurysmal type

Acquired

Secondary to trauma, surgery, inflammation, renal cell carcinoma.

INFERIOR VENA CAVA PATHOLOGY

Congenital
- Infrahepatic interruption: failure of union of the hepatic veins and right subcardial (either azygos or hemiazygos continuation).
- Double IVC (<3%)
- Membranous obstruction may simulate infrahepatic interruption.

IVC DILATION
- In young people look for changes in respiration (collapse).
- Evaluate retrograde flow from right atrium into IVC.

Causes
- Right ventricular failure
- CHD
- Constrictive pericarditis
- Tricuspid disease
- Right atrial tumor
- Hepatomegaly

TUMOR OR THROMBUS
Patients may have internal echoes in IVC secondary to renal tumor, portal hypertension, or Budd Chiari.

IVC OBSTRUCTION
1. Thin membrane at level of entrance to right atrium.
2. Absent segment of IVC without characteristic conical narrowing.
3. Complete obstruction secondary to thrombosis.

TUMORS IN THE IVC
- Hepatic portion: IVC compresses.
- Posterior caudate lobe and RLL: tumor may elevate IVC.
- Localized liver mass produces posterior lateral or medial displacement of IVC.

- Mid or pancreatic portion.
- Abnormality of right renal artery, right kidney, or nodes may elevate IVC.
- Lower small bowel segment: lumbar spine anomalies, nodes, may elevate IVC.

RENAL VEIN OBSTRUCTION

- Complication seen in dehydrated or septic infants.
- May be seen in adults with multiple renal anomalies.
- Associated with maternal diabetes and transient hypertension.
- IVP shows absent or faintly visualized kidney.
- Sonography used to exclude hydro and confirm the palpable renal mass or multicystic kidney causing the obstruction.

RENAL VEIN ENLARGEMENT

Left renal vein obstruction.

Causes

- Carcinoma of pancreas, lung, or lymphoma, thrombosis, or retroperitoneal tumor

Sonography

If following patterns are present on sonography, renal vein thrombosis may be present:
1. Direct visualization of thrombi in renal vein and IVC.
2. Demonstration of renal vein dilated proximal to point of occlusion.
3. Loss of normal renal structure.
4. Increased renal size in acute phase.
5. Doppler shows decreased or no flow.

IVC FILTERS

- Most common origin of pulmonary emboli is venous thrombosis from lower extremities.

- Used to prevent recurrent embolization in patients who cannot tolerate anticoagulants.
- Preferred location is in iliac bifurcation, below renal veins.
- Some filters can migrate or perforate the wall, producing a retroperitoneal bleed.

DISTORTION OF THE IVC

Causes
- Extrinsic retroperitoneal mass
- Hepatic neoplasm, pancreatic mass
- IVC tumor

PANCREAS

NORMAL PANCREAS SIZE: Under 2.5 cm thick, 12 cm long.
PANCREAS DUCT: 2 mm.

ANNULAR PANCREAS

Lab/Symptoms
- GI symptoms.
- Enlarged stomach and duodenal bulb secondary to pancreatic constriction.
- More frequent in males.

Sonography
- Pancreatic tissue surrounds the second portion of the duodenum.

CYSTADENOMA

Lab/Symptoms

- More frequent in middle-age women.
- Abdominal pain and increased amylase

Sonography

- Usually anechoic, may have septa, thick walls.
- Differential would include pseudocyst.

PANCREATIC CARCINOMA

Lab/Symptoms

- Painless jaundice if mass constricts common bile duct (Courvoisier's sign), weight loss, back pain.

Sonography

- Focal mass with irregular borders, hypo to isoechoic.
- May cause obstruction of pancreatic duct.

PANCREATITIS (ACUTE)

- Associated with alcohol abuse or biliary disease.
- Trauma or viral infections may be cause, especially in children.

Lab/Symptoms

- Upper abdominal pain radiating to back.
- Nausea and vomiting.
- Ileus.
- Increased serum amylase and lipase.

Sonography

- Focal to diffuse enlargement of the pancreas, hypoechoic texture, irregular borders.
- Look for pseudocyst formation, or extrapancreatic fluid collections in lesser sac, anterior pararenal space, or perivascular area.

PSEUDOCYST

- Found in 10% of patients with pancreatitis.
- Results from contained collections of pancreatic secretions and debris.
- May become infected leading to abscess.
- Usually occur in the lesser sac behind the stomach of the left anterior pararenal space.

Lab/Symptoms

- Usually presents with pancreatitis.
- Persistent abdominal pain, radiating to back.
- Elevated amylase.

Sonography

- Sterile collection of pancreatic enzymes that has walled off to fill available space around collection.
- Borders are usually smooth, with debris along posterior border.
- Posterior enhancement.
- Found anywhere in abdomen or pelvis.
- If large, may displace normal organs surrounding mass.
- May spontaneously drain into stomach, duodenum, or bowel.

PANCREATITIS (CHRONIC)

- Results from recurrent acute or subacute pancreatitis leading to destruction of the gland.
- Alcohol most common cause.

Lab/Symptoms

- Previous problems with acute pancreatitis.
- Constant midepigastric pain radiating to back.
- May have mild jaundice, nausea and vomiting.
- May lead to diabetes.

Sonography

- Gland atrophy and irregular outline.
- Calculi in the duct or its branches.
- Dilation of the duct to greater than 2 mm diameter.
- Focal gland enlargement usually involving head of pancreas.
- Calcification in a focal mass favors pancreatitis over tumor.

LIVER

NORMAL LIVER SIZE: Longitudinal measurement from diaphragm to right edge of liver is 15 cm.

Sonography
- Liver parenchyma is homogeneous.

BLOOD AND BILE FLOW PATTERNS
- Portal veins carry blood from bowel to liver.
- Hepatic veins drain blood from liver to IVC.
- Hepatic arteries carry oxygenated blood from aorta to liver.
- Bile ducts transport bile (manufactured by the liver) to the duodenum.
- Caudate lobe is the only lobe that receives blood from the portal and hepatic artery.

HEPATIC SEGMENTS
   RIGHT LOBE: Anterior and posterior segments.
   LEFT LOBE: Medial and lateral segments.

CAUDATE LOBE: Posterior portion is between fossa of the IVC and fissure of the ligamentum venosum.

HEPATIC VEINS
RIGHT HEPATIC VEIN: Enters right lateral aspect of IVC.
MID HEPATIC VEIN: Enters anterior or right anterior surface of IVC.
LEFT HEPATIC VEIN: Enters left/anterior surface of IVC.
- Hepatic veins run in the interlobar fissures and separate the functional lobes (portal veins run within the segments and between the hepatic veins).

FUNCTIONAL DIVISIONS OF LIVER
PURPOSE: To separate liver into component parts according to blood supply and biliary drainage so that one component can be removed in event of tumor or trauma.

LIVER FUNCTION
- Secretes bile.
- Removes nutrients from blood.
- Converts glucose to glycogen and stores it.
- Stores iron and vitamins.
- Converts excess amino acids to fatty acids.
- Metabolism of proteins, fats, carbohydrates.
- Manufactures many plasma proteins found in blood.
- Detoxifies many drugs and poisons that enter body.
- Phagocytizes bacteria and worn out red blood cells.

HEPATIC TERMINOLOGY
BARE AREA: Area where the peritoneal reflections from the liver onto the diaphragm leave an irregular triangle of liver without peritoneal covering.

CORONARY LIGAMENT: Peritoneal reflections around the bare area.

HEPATORENAL LIGAMENT: Caudal part of coronary ligament reflected onto diaphragm and right kidney.

HEPATORENAL POUCH or POUCH OF MORISON: Area below the hepatorenal ligament bounded by the liver, kidney, colon, and duodenum (potential site for fluid collection).

SUBPHRENIC SPACE: Space between liver or spleen and diaphragm (common site for abscess or fluid collection).

LESSER SAC: Enclosed portion of peritoneal space behind liver and stomach.

- *RIGHT*: Kidney and liver.
- *LEFT*: Kidney and spleen.
- Liver is superior to lesser sac.
- Transverse colon is inferior to lesser sac.
- Stomach is anterior to lesser sac.
- Pancreas and great vessels are posterior to lesser sac.

SUBPHRENIC SPACES

RIGHT AND LEFT ANTERIOR SUBPHRENIC SPACES: Lie between diaphragm and liver on each side of falciform ligament.

RIGHT POSTERIOR SUBPHRENIC SPACE: Lies amid right lobe of liver, right kidney, and right colic flexure.

RIGHT EXTRAPERITONEAL SPACE: Lies between layers of coronary ligament between liver and diaphragm.

LIVER FOSSAE

THREE IMPORTANT FOSSAE: IVC, right kidney, gallbladder.

Hepatic Lobe Blood Supply and Drainage

Lobe	Supplied by	Drained by
Right lobe	Right portal vein Right hepatic artery	Right hepatic vein and right bile duct
Left lobe	Left portal vein Left hepatic artery	Left hepatic vein and left bile duct
Caudate lobe	Right or left portal vein Right or left hepatic artery	Variable or both

Anatomic Structures Useful for Dividing and Identifying Hepatic Segments

Structure	Location	Usefulness
Right hepatic vein	Right intersegmental fissure	Divides cephalic aspect of anterior and posterior segments of right hepatic lobe and courses between the anterior and posterior branches of right portal vein
Middle hepatic vein	Main lobar fissure	Separates right and left lobes
Left hepatic vein	Left intersegmental fissure	Divides cephalic aspects of medial and lateral segments of left lobe
Right portal vein (anterior)	Intrasegmental in anterior segment of right hepatic lobe	Courses centrally in anterior segment of right hepatic lobe

Table continued on next page.

Anatomic Structures Useful for Dividing and Identifying Hepatic Segments—cont'd

Structure	Location	Usefulness
Right portal vein (posterior)	Intrasegmental in posterior segment of right hepatic lobe	Courses centrally in posterior segment of right hepatic lobe
Left portal vein (initial)	Courses anterior to caudate lobe	Separates caudate lobe posterior from medial segment of left lobe anterior
Left portal vein (ascending)	Turns anterior in left intersegmental fissure	Divides medial and lateral segment of left lobe
IVC fossa	Posterior aspect of main lobar fissure	Separates right and left hepatic lobes
GB fossa	Main lobar fissure	Separates right and left hepatic lobes
Ligamentum teres	Left intersegmental fissure	Divides caudal aspect of left hepatic lobe into medial and lateral segments
Fissure of ligamentum venosum	Left anterior margin of caudate lobe	Separates caudate lobe from medial and lateral segments of left lobe

LIVER PATHOLOGY

FATTY LIVER (DIFFUSE DISEASE)

Common Causes

- Alcoholic liver.
- Diabetes mellitus.
- Obesity.
- Protein-calorie malnutrition.
- Chronic illness (TB, CHF, inflammatory bowel).
- Severe hepatitis.
- Steroids.
- Parenteral nutrition.

Lab/Symptoms

- May have influenza-like symptoms.
- Loss of appetite.
- Nausea.
- Vomiting.
- Fatigue.
- RUQ pain.
- Increased SGOT, SGPT, bilirubin.
- May be jaundiced.

Sonography of Diffuse Fatty Liver Disease

- Increased echogenicity.
- Increased attenuation.
- Irregular borders of intrahepatic vessels.
- Hepatomegaly.

- Sonographic discrimination between fatty liver and cirrhosis may be difficult.

Sonography of Focal Fatty Liver Disease
- Patchy distribution.
- Nonspherical.
- Poor margins.
- Fan shaped.
- No mass effect (nondisplaced portal vasculature).

HEPATITIS

Lab/Symptoms
- Elevated liver enzymes (SGOT, SGPT—but falls rapidly after several days).
- Increased bilirubin.
- Exposure to type A or B hepatitis; most common liver disease.

Sonography of Acute Hepatitis
- Nonspecific findings, variable parenchyma pattern.
- Decreased echogenicity if severe.
- Increased brightness of portal venous walls.
- Hepatomegaly

Sonography of Chronic Hepatitis
Same as acute except:
- Coarsening of echoes.
- Increased echogenicity.
- Decreased visualization of vessels.

HEMOCHROMATOSIS

Lab/Symptoms

- Excessive iron deposition especially in liver, spleen, lymph nodes, pancreas, gastrointestinal tract, kidneys, heart, endocrine glands.
- Leads to cirrhosis and portal hypertension.
- Primary and secondary forms.
- Predisposed to hepatoma (secondary to cirrhosis).

Sonography

- Does not show specific findings, i.e., hepatomegaly with increased parenchymal echoes, cirrhosis, or hepatoma may be present.

GLYCOGEN STORAGE DISEASE

Lab/Symptoms

- Appearance is variable, depends on type of disease.
- Increased incidence of adenomas with Type I glycogen storage disease.

Sonography

- Hepatomegaly.
- Increased echogenicity.
- Increased attenuation.
- Adenoma: round; homogeneous, if small; may be inhomogeneous if large; increased transmission.

VON GIERKE'S DISEASE

Lab/Symptoms

- Type I glycogen storage disease is most prevalent kind.
- Activity of the enzyme glucose-6-phosphate is impaired, preventing glycogenolysis and release of glucose.

Sonography

- Hepatomegaly
- Fatty infiltrated liver.
- Associated with hepatic adenomas, focal nodular hyperplasia.

CIRRHOSIS

Lab/Symptoms

- Increased serum and urine bilirubin.
- Increased ALP, AST.
- Alcohol abuse.
- Necrosis of liver tissue.

CLINICAL

- Acute[m]nausea, vomiting.
- Chronic[m]jaundice, ascites, GI bleeding.

Sonography

- Increased echogenicity.
- Increased attenuation.
- Hepatomegaly, splenomegaly (acute).
- Decreased liver, spleen size (chronic).
- Decreased vascular markings.
- Ascites.
- Nodularity.
- Accentuation of fissures.
- Regenerating nodules (isoechoic).
- Hepatoma.
- Fibrosis may cause normal parenchyma to be hypoechoic.
- Evidence for portal hypertension, varices, reversal of flow.

BUDD CHIARI SYNDROME

Lab/Symptoms

- Results from obstruction to hepatic venous drainage.
- Classification:
  1. Occlusion of IVC.
  2. Primary occlusion of hepatic veins.
  3. Occlusion of small centrilobular veins.

Causes

- Idiopathic.
- Polycythemia vera.
- Contraceptives.
- Tumors (hepatic, renal, adrenal, IVC).
- Fibrous webs in IVC.
- Pregnancy.
- Trauma.

Sonography

- Enlargement of caudate lobe.
- Atrophy of other lobes, inhomogeneity.
- Thrombus in hepatic veins and/or IVC.
- Collaterals.
- Ascites.

FOCAL DISEASES OF LIVER

Focal fatty infiltration, abscess, cysts, hematoma, primary tumor, metastases.

ABSCESS
PYOGENIC: Most common.

Lab/Symptoms
Source of infection:
1. Cholangitis.
2. Portal pyemia secondary to appendicitis, diverticulitis, inflammatory disease, colitis.
3. Direct spread from contiguous organ (gallbladder).
4. Trauma with direct contamination.
5. Infarction (postembolization, sickle cell).

Multiple in 50% to 70% of patients; right posterior lobe of liver most frequently involved.

Sonography
- Hypoechoic.
- Round margins.
- Acoustic enhancement.
- Variable amount of debris.
- May have fluid level.
- If gas is present, may be hyperechoic with shadowing and reverberation.

Sonography of Amebic Abscess

- Appearance variable.
- Homogeneous, hypoechoic with layer of debris.
- Well-defined, smooth thin walls.
- Older lesion shows walls more hyperechoic.
- Acoustic enhancement.
- May have disruption of diaphragm.
- Resolution with therapy (6 weeks to 2 years).
- Aspiration drainage.

HEPATIC CANDIDIASIS

Lab/Symptoms

- Infection by fungi.
- Hepatomegaly.
- Occurs in immunocompromised hosts.

Sonography

- Multiple small hypoechoic masses with echogenic centers (target sign).

ECHINOCOCCAL DISEASE

Lab/Symptoms

- Cyst stage of infection by parasite tapeworm.
- Liver most commonly affected.
- Found in sheep raising countries.

Sonography

- Large cysts.
- Thick walls.
- Septations frequent.

- Daughter cysts (small cysts internally tangent to mother cyst).
- Floating membranes.
- Calcifications (walls).

HEPATIC CYSTS

Lab/Symptoms

- May present asymptomatic.
- If cyst is large, with palpable mass.
- LFTs are normal.

Sonography

- Well-demarcated, anechoic mass.
- Smooth walled.
- Enhanced posterior transmission.
- Multiple or solitary.
- May contain septa.

HEPATIC TUMORS

BENIGN: Cavernous hemangioma, focal nodular hyperplasia, hepatic adenoma, biliary cystadenoma.

MALIGNANT: Hepatoma, biliary cystadenocarcinoma, metastases, cholangiocarcinoma.

CAVERNOUS HEMANGIOMA

Lab/Symptoms

- Most common benign tumor of liver in females.
- Asymptomatic.
- 4.5% may bleed.
- Subcapsular.
- Right lobe.
- 20% pedunculated.

Sonography
- Most are hyperechoic.
- Large hemangiomas may have mixed pattern due to necrosis.
- Acoustic enhancement.

Differential Diagnosis
- Metastatic disease.
- Hepatoma.
- Focal nodular hyperplasia.
- Adenoma.

FOCAL NODULAR HYPERPLASIA (FNH)

Lab/Symptoms
- Not related to contraception but increased bleed in patients taking birth control pill.
- 2:1 female.
- No malignant potential.
- Right lobe over left.
- 20% multiple.
- Most are subcapsular, some pedunculated, most central scar.

Sonography
- Well-defined.
- Subcapsular mass.
- Isoechoic or hyperechoic.
- Central stellate group of echoes.

HEPATIC ADENOMA

Lab/Symptoms
- Related to contraceptives, androgens, steroids.
- Increased incidence of hemorrhage.

- Female over males.
- Increased incidence in patients with Von Gierke's disease.

Sonography

- Usually hyperechoic.
- May have central hypoechoic areas due to hemorrhage.
- Fluid in peritoneal cavity if ruptured.

METASTATIC DISEASE

Lab/Symptoms

- 25-50% of patients dying of cancer have metastases to liver.
- Most frequent primary sites are colon, lung, breast, pancreas.
- CT and ultrasound more sensitive than nuclear medicine.

Sonography

- Sensitive to detect small lesions.
- Primary imaging modality.
- Most metastases are hypoechoic.
- Hyperechoic metastases seen with colon cancer and pancreatic cancer (bulls-eye or target sign).
- Calcifications, especially with colon metastases.

HEPATOCELLULAR CARCINOMA

Lab/Symptoms

- Comprises 90% of primary liver malignancies.
- Men over women.
- Causes: cirrhosis, chronic hepatitis, carcinogens.
- Portal vein invasion in 25% to 40% of cases.
- Hepatic vein invasion in 16%

Sonography

- Variable:
  1. Discrete lesions: Solitary or multiple, usually hypoechoic or hyperechoic, may have halo.
  2. Diffuse: Inhomogeneity throughout, no distinct masses.
  3. Combination.
- Cannot tell hepatoma versus metastases.
- Thrombus in portal, hepatic veins, IVC.

HEPATIC TRAUMA

Lab/Symptoms

- Third most common organ injured after spleen and kidney.
- 3% of trauma patients.
- Frequently associated with other organs injured.
- Need for surgery determined by size of laceration.
- Right lobe most frequent.
- May be small laceration, large, or large with hematoma, subcapsular hemorrhage, capsular disruption.

Sonography

- Not used as frequently as computed tomography.
- Subcapsular hematomas:
  - Anechoic.
  - Hyperechoic or septated lenticular, or curvilinear.
- Internal hepatic hematomas:
  - Hyperechoic first 24 hours.
  - Hypoechoic thereafter with complex interior.
  - Septations with internal echoes in 1 to 4 weeks.
- Fluid in abdomen.
- Ultrasound difficult with small laceration in dome of right lobe.

GALLBLADDER AND BILIARY SYSTEM

BILIARY SYSTEM

Right and left hepatic ducts emerge from right lobe liver in porta hepatis to form the common hepatic duct. Hepatic duct passes caudally and medially and runs parallel to portal vein.

COMMON HEPATIC DUCT: 4 mm in diameter, joined by cystic duct to form common bile duct.

CYSTIC DUCT: Connects neck of gallbladder with common hepatic duct to form common bile duct in right free edge of lesser omentum.

COMMON BILE DUCT: 6 mm or less in diameter.

- First part lies in right free edge of lesser omentum.
- Second part lies posterior to 1st part of duodenum.
- Third part lies in groove on posterior surface of head of pancreas.
- Ends at wall of second part of duodenum.
- Joined by main pancreatic duct and both go through ampulla of Vater into duodenal wall surrounded by circle muscle fiber sphincter of Oddi.
- Proximal portion of common bile duct is lateral to hepatic artery and anterior to portal vein.
- Duct becomes more posterior after it descends behind duodenal bulb and enters pancreas.
- Distal part is parallel to anterior wall of IVC.
- Ducts follow same course as portal veins and hepatic artery.
- Encased in common sheath to form portal triad.

GALLBLADDER

Normal Gallbladder Size

- 3 cm transverse diameter and 7 to 10 cm long
- Divided into fundus, body, and neck.
- Arterial supply by cystic artery (branch of right hepatic artery).
- Venous drainage is via cystic vein that drains directly into portal system.

Sonography

- Anechoic ovoid structure in right upper quadrant.

GALLBLADDER FUNCTION

Stores bile and enzymes secreted into duodenum primarily when fat is present.

ADENOMYOMATOSIS

Lab/Symptoms

- Asymptomatic.
- Adenomyomatous hyperplasia may be diffuse.
- Localized or segmental.

Sonography

- Diffuse or segmental gallbladder wall thickening.
- Intramural diverticula with anechoic or echogenic foci.
- Reverberation artifacts.

CHOLEDOCHAL CYST

Anomalous insertion of common bile duct into pancreatic duct permitting reflux of pancreatic juice into bile duct leading to cholangitis and dilatation.

Lab/Symptoms

- More common in females and orientals.
- Pain.

- Intermittent jaundice.
- Palpable mass.

Sonography
- Large cystic mass in porta hepatis separate from gallbladder.
- Dilated common hepatic duct or common bile duct entering directly into mass.
- Calculi may be present within the cyst.

Differential Diagnosis
- Hepatic cyst.
- Pancreatic pseudocyst.
- Hepatic artery aneurysm.
- Perforation of the extrahepatic ducts.

CHOLELITHIASIS

Lab/Symptoms
- RUQ pain.
- Positive Murphy's sign.
- More common in females.
- Nausea and vomiting.

Sonography of Cholelithiasis
- Echodense mass within the gallbladder.
- Acoustic "clean" shadow posterior.
- Density should move when patient changes position.
- "Floating" gallstones secondary to thick bile.
- "Packed bag" seen when gallbladder is filled with stones.
- "Porcelain" gallbladder when walls are calcified.

Sonography of Choledocholithiasis
- Obstruction.
- Hydrops develops with obstruction to cystic duct.

- In calculous obstruction, gallbladder may be small.
- Stone projects as curvilinear with strong acoustic shadow.

Sonography of Sludge

- Low level, finely stippled echoes along posterior wall.
- No acoustic shadow present.
- May assume unusual shape and not change with position due to thick bile.

CHOLECYSTITIS (ACUTE)

Lab/Symptoms

- More common in females.
- RUQ pain radiating to right shoulder.
- Fever.
- Nausea.
- Vomiting.
- Jaundice may be present.
- Intolerance to fatty food.

Causes

- Chemical irritation by concentrated bile.
- Bacterial infection.
- Pancreatic reflux.

Sonography of Cholecystitis (Acute)

- Enlarged gallbladder (>5 cm).
- Round or oval shape.
- Thickened gallbladder wall with edema.
- Pericholecystic abscess formation.
- Vascular congestion.
- Pus in lumen and gallstones seen in empyema of the gallbladder.

- Necrosis of gallbladder with ulcerations seen in gangrene of gallbladder may result in pericholecystic fluid.

Sonography of Cholecystitis (Chronic)

- Contracted gallbladder.
- Usually gallstones are present.
- Wall is thickened.

Sonography of Emphysematous Cholecystitis

- Acoustic shadowing from gas/air in the gallbladder wall/lumen.

GALLBLADDER CARCINOMA

Lab/Symptoms

- More common in the elderly female.
- Common site is in fundus and neck.
- Patient may be asymptomatic or present with loss of appetite.
- Nausea and vomiting.
- Intolerance to fatty foods.
- Belching.
- Jaundice is present when there is infiltration of biliary ducts and extension into the liver.

Sonography

- Gallstones may be present.
- May see calcification in gallbladder wall.
- Infiltrating type: poorly defined area of diffuse thickening and induration in the gallbladder wall.
- Fungating type: grows into the lumen as irregular cauliflower mass invading the wall.
- May extend into liver, cystic duct, and adjacent bile ducts.
- Mass appears solid with irregular borders.

SPLEEN AND RETROPERITONEAL SPACE

NORMAL SPLENIC SIZE: 9 to 12 cm in longitudinal decubitus.

Sonography of the Normal Spleen

- Homogeneous parenchymal tissue with internal vascular channels for splenic artery and vein.

FUNCTION OF SPLEEN

- Active in blood formation during initial part of fetal life.
- Role in the defense mechanism of the body.
- Role in pigment and lipid metabolism.
- Production of lymphocytes and plasma cells.
- Production of antibodies.
- Storage of iron and other metabolites.

SPLENIC CYST

Lab/Symptoms

- More common in females
- Asymptomatic.

Sonography

- Hypoechoic or anechoic foci.
- Well-defined walls.
- Increased through transmission.

GRANULOMATOUS INFECTION

Lab/Symptoms

- May be secondary to acute or chronic infection.

Sonography

- Splenomegaly
- Diffuse hypoechogenicity.

INFARCT OR RUPTURE

Lab/Symptoms

- Occurs secondary to septic emboli and local thromboses in patients with pancreatitis, subacute bacterial endocarditis, leukemia, lymphomatous disorders, or sickle cell anemia.

Sonography

- May see localized hypoechoic area (fresh infarct).
- Healed infarct shows as wedge-shaped lesion.

RETROPERITONEAL CAVITY

RETROPERITONEAL SPACE: Area between posterior portion of parietal peritoneum and post abdominal wall muscles.

- Extends from diaphragm to pelvis.
- Lateral boundaries: extends to extraperitoneal fat planes within transversalis fascia.
- Medial boundaries: space encloses the great vessels.
- Divided into three areas:
  1. Perinephric space.
  2. Anterior paranephric space.
  3. Posterior paranephric space.

LYMPHADENOPATHY

- 40% of lymphomas are Hodgkin's disease; remainder is non-Hodgkin's.
- Need to evaluate paraortic and paracaval adenopathy, metastatic spread to liver, spleen, kidneys.

LYMPHOMA (NON-HODGKIN'S)

Lab/Symptoms

- >40% have mesenteric disease.

Sonography of Non-Hodgkin's Lymphoma

- 40% have paraortic nodal involvement.
- Nodes appear hypoechoic to anechoic with good transmission.
- Nodes may be very large.
- May see mantle-like plaque of tumor along vertebral body.
- May see organ compression or obscuration of outlines of paraortic structures (silhouette sign).

Sonography of Hodgkin's Lymphoma

- 25% have paraortic nodal involvement.

Sonography of Burkitt's Lymphoma:

- Abdominal masses tend to be large and solitary.
- Mass may be found in pelvis, upper abdomen, and retroperitoneum.
- Increased incidence of ileocecal, mesenteric, or ovarian involvement.
- Terminal ileum common site.
- Tumor may appear lucent to hyperechoic.
- Mass is well defined, sharply marginated, and homogeneous.

RETROPERITONEAL MASSES

Sonography

- *Liposarcoma*: Echo-reflective, irregularly thickened wall, complex echo pattern.
- *Sarcoma*: Increased or decreased internal echoes or echodense central area with hypoechoic periphery.
- *Leiomyosarcomas*: Undergo necrosis and cystic degeneration.
- *Fibrosarcomas* and *rhabdomyosarcomas*: Invasive and infiltrate into muscle and adjoining soft tissue.
- *Teratomas*: Heterogeneously mixed with solid areas, calcification, and cystic spaces.

RETROPERITONEAL FIBROSIS

Lab/Symptoms

- Back.
- Flank, or abdominal pain with weight loss, nausea and vomiting, and malaise.
- Palpable mass may be present.
- Hypertension common.
- More frequent in middle-age males.

Sonography

- Large, bulky mass with ill-defined, irregular margins.
- May show as a flat, large mass with smooth margins extending from pelvis into abdomen.
- Mass may be anechoic to hypoechoic.
- Anterior margin easier to delineate than posterior border.

KIDNEY

NORMAL RENAL SIZE: 9-12 cm long; 2-3 cm thick; and 4-5 cm wide.

- Surrounded by fibrous capsule called *true capsule*.
- This is closely applied to renal cortex.
- Outside is covering of *perinephric fat*.
- *Perinephric fascia* surrounds this fat and encloses kidney and adrenal gland.
- *Renal fascia*: perinephric fascia surrounds the true capsule and perinephric fat.

Sonography

- Cortex: Homogeneously echogenic with low-level echoes similar in density to the liver parenchyma.
- Medulla: Pyramids are hypoechoic.
- Arcuate vessels: At corticomedullary junction are high-level echoes; serve as a marker for the evaluation of cortical thickness.
- Columns of Bertin: Cortical tissue extending into space between the adjacent pyramids.
- Renal sinus: Contains collecting system, renal vessels, lymphatics, fat, fibrous tissue. Appears as ovoid intense echo collection in kidney on long axis and rounded echodense area on transverse.

URETER
THREE CONSTRICTIONS:
1. Where it joins the kidney at the hilum (UPJ).
2. Where it crosses the pelvic brim.
3. Where it pierces the posterior/lateral bladder wall.

ANGIOMYOLIPOMA

Lab/Symptoms

- Uncommon benign renal fatty tumor (intermixed with smooth muscle cells and aggregates of thick-walled blood vessels.
- Usually unilateral, may be multiple.
- More common in females and in the right kidney.
- 60% to 80% with tuberous sclerosis have these lesions.
- Usually present asymptomatic.
- May have hemorrhage within the lesion or in the retroperitoneum (flank or abdominal pain/shock).

Sonography

- Hyperechoic lesion (due to high fat content).
- Multiple nonfat interfaces.

- Heterogeneous cellular architecture and/or numerous vessels.
- Mixed pattern suggests hemorrhage and necrosis.

RENAL ADENOMA

Lab/Symptoms
- Asymptomatic.

Sonography
- Small lesion (<3 cm).
- Hypoechoic.

RENAL CYST

Lab/Symptoms
- May be asymptomatic, usually incidental finding.

Sonography of Simple Renal Cyst
- Cyst arises in renal cortex.
- Usually single.
- Anechoic, well-defined, with acoustic enhancement.

Sonography of Pararenal Cyst
- Cyst in hilum of the kidney.
- No communication with collecting system.

Sonography of Multiloculated Cyst
- Large tumor with multiple fluid-filled masses.
- Masses separated by highly echogenic septations with normal renal tissue in rest of kidney.

Sonography of Multicystic Dysplastic Kidney
- Common cause of abdominal mass in newborn.
- Left kidney affected twice as often as the right.
- Cysts of varying sizes.

- No connection between adjacent multiple cysts.
- Absence of identifiable renal sinus.
- Absence of renal parenchyma surrounding cysts.
- Presence of eccentric echogenic areas.

Sonography of Infantile Polycystic Kidney Disease

- Poor definition of renal sinus, medulla, and cortex.
- Diffuse echogenicity.
- Irregular cortical surface.

Sonography of Adult Polycystic Kidney Disease

- Enlarged kidneys.
- Discrete cysts in cortical region.
- Renal contour poorly demarcated from surrounding tissue.
- Associated cysts may be found in liver, pancreas, spleen.
- Usually bilateral.

RENAL CARCINOMA

Lab/Symptoms

- Lesion is seen in the older male.
- Costovertebral angle pain.
- Mass.
- Hematuria.
- Metastases common (lungs, bones, nodes, liver, adrenal, and brain; 10% to 15% to opposite kidney).

Sonography

- Mass is more or less echogenic than normal kidney parenchyma.
- No acoustic enhancement posterior.
- Irregular margins.
- No direct correlation between echogenicity and vascularity.
- Inhomogeneity due to hemorrhage, necrosis, or cystic degeneration.

- Examine contralateral kidney for extension of tumor.
- Examine inferior vena cava, paraortic area, and renal vein for tumor extension.

ACUTE GLOMERULONEPHRITIS

Lab/Symptoms
- More common in younger males.
- Oliguria.
- Hematuria.
- Hypertension.
- Fatigue.
- Nausea and vomiting.
- Fever.
- Recent infection.

Sonography
- Pyramids well-visualized secondary to edema.
- Enlarged kidneys.
- Increased echogenicity of cortex.

CHRONIC GLOMERULONEPHRITIS

Lab/Symptoms
- Common cause of renal failure.
- Oliguria, polyuria, hypertension.

Sonography
- Small renal size.
- Increased cortical echogenicity.

HYDRONEPHROSIS

Lab/Symptoms
- May be asymptomatic.

- May be associated with renal obstruction.

Sonography
- Fluid-filled renal pelvis and calyceal system.
- Look for site of obstruction; follow course of ureter into bladder.
- Calculi would project as echogenic reflection with shadowing.
- Postvoid images to see if hydronephrosis disappears.
- Bladder jets.

LUPUS NEPHRITIS

Lab/Symptoms
- Females (20-40 years).
- Renal disease.
- Vasculitis.
- Hematologic abnormalities.

Sonography
- Increased echogenicity of renal cortex.
- Renal size increased or normal.

NEPHROLITHIASIS

Lab/Symptoms
- Increased calcium salts in the renal parenchyma, more in males.
- May present with a variety of conditions (hyperparathyroid, medullary sponge kidney).

Sonography
- Echogenic foci within the renal cortex, along the corticomedullary junction.
- In medullary nephrocalcinosis there are focal areas of increased echogenicity corresponding to the renal pyramids (no acoustic shadow).

PYELONEPHRITIS, ACUTE

Lab/Symptoms

- Mostly females.
- Dysuria.
- Frequency.
- Urgency.
- Chills.
- Fever.
- Malaise.
- Back pain.
- Tender.
- Bacterial infection.

Sonography

- Normal to enlarged kidney.
- Increased anechoic corticomedullary area with multiple scattered low-level echoes (abscess collections).
- May have hydronephrosis.

PYELONEPHRITIS, CHRONIC

Lab/Symptoms

- May be asymptomatic.
- Proteinuria.
- Chronic UTI.
- Hypotensive.
- Dysuria.
- Frequency.
- Polyuria.

Sonography

- Focal or multifocal process with loss of renal parenchyma.
- Retraction of one or more calyces.
- Decrease in renal size.
- Increased echoes in involved area of medulla and cortex.

RENAL FAILURE

Lab/Symptoms

- Reduction in renal function associated with an increase in serum creatinine.

Sonography of Acute Renal Failure

- Renal size normal or enlarged.
- Medulla well seen (edema).
- Exclude hydronephrosis.

Sonography of Chronic Renal Failure

- Renal size may be decreased.
- Renal parenchymal pattern more echogenic than the liver.

SINUS LIPOMATOSIS

Lab/Symptoms

- Common in older patients.
- Linked to obesity.
- Parenchymal atrophy or destruction.
- May have chronic calculous disease and inflammation.

Sonography

- May show renal enlargement.
- Renal sinus fat is increased.

WILMS' TUMOR

Lab/Symptoms

- Most common solid renal tumor in children under eight (peak at 3 years).
- May present with large asymptomatic flank mass.
- Uncommon to have abdominal pain, fever, hematuria, or anorexia.
- Hypertension is present.

Sonography of Wilms' Tumor

- Varies from hypoechoic to moderately echogenic.
- Irregular anechoic areas seen corresponding to central necrosis and hemorrhage.
- Sharply marginated with compressed renal tissue.
- Examine contralateral kidney, renal vein, and IVC for tumor invasion.

Sonography of Nephroblastoma

- Multicystic mass of varying sizes.
- Subcapsular and parenchymal hypoechoic areas.
- Nephromegaly with decreased parenchymal echoes.
- May be difficult to separate from Wilms' tumor
- Heterogeneous with irregular hyperechoic areas intermixed with less echogenic areas.

XANTHOGRANULOMATOUS PYELONEPHRITIS

Lab/Symptoms

- Long-term urinary tract infection.
- Malaise.
- Flank pain.
- Weight loss.
- Urinary tract infection.

Sonography
- Ultrasound pattern varies with level of infection.
- *Diffuse*: Parenchyma replaced by multiple circular, apparently fluid-filled masses that surround the central echo complex.
- Masses correspond to debris-filled dilated calyces and/or foci of parenchymal destruction.
- Kidney enlarged.
- Echogenicity of masses dependent on amount of debris and necrosis within them.
- Echogenic stone may be difficult to define.
- *Segmental*: One or more masses surrounding a single calyx that contains a calculus.
- Masses may be hypoechoic or anechoic.

RENAL TRANSPLANT
Renal Transplant ATN
- Most common cause of acute posttransplant renal failure.
- Increased creatinine.
- Low urine output.
- Renal sinus may show decreased echogenicity.

Renal Transplant Graft Rupture
- Occurs secondary to acute rejection.
- Tachycardia, hypotension, oliguria, decreased hematocrit, pain, tenderness, and swelling.
- Hemorrhage occurs along lateral border of kidney.

Renal Transplant Obstruction
- Degree of dilation may be influenced more by amount of bladder distention.

- Look for obstruction or stricture at ureterovesical junction, torsion, extrinsic compression, ureteral necrosis, or blood clots.

Renal Transplant Rejection
- Most common cause of renal failure after the first week.
- Fever, graft tenderness, and oliguria.
- Acute: Increased renal size (edema, congestion).
- Cortical ischemia: Focal edema, hemorrhage, infarction (decrease in parenchymal echogenicity).
- Enlarged pyramids.
- Loss of corticomedullary junction definition.
- Decreased amplitude of renal sinus echoes.
- Perirenal fluid.

Renal Transplant Lymphocele
- Lymph drains into peritoneal cavity.
- Causes decrease in renal function.
- Painless swelling over renal area.
- Presents as well-defined anechoic to hypoechoic cystic area.
- Septations may be present.

Renal Transplant Urinoma
- Urine leak may be serious complication.
- Look for defect at ureteropelvic, ureteroureter, or ureterovesical anastomosis.
- May present with decreased urine output, pain, swelling over transplant.
- Hypoechoic mass with internal septation near lower pole.
- Hydronephrosis.

ADRENAL

Sonography
- Hypoechoic structure surrounded by echogenic fat.
- Well imaged in the fetal and neonatal stage.

ADRENAL ADENOMA

Lab/Symptoms
- Endocrine abnormalities, frequently nonsecreting.

Sonography
- Incidental finding.
- Bilateral.
- Size varies.
- May be encapsulated, solid, hypoechoic.
- May have calcification.
- May be multiple.

ADRENAL CYST

Lab/Symptoms
- Asymptomatic.
- May be hypertensive.

Sonography
- Anechoic.
- Posterior displacement of superior pole of kidney.
- May calcify.
- May be heterogeneous with low level echoes secondary to hemorrhage.

ADRENAL HEMORRHAGE

Lab/Symptoms
- More common in neonates.
- Present with flank mass, jaundice, increased bilirubin.

Sonography
- Complex mass superior to upper pole kidney.
- May see calcifications.
- May follow to see regression of bleed.

ADRENAL HYPERPLASIA

Lab/Symptoms
- Obesity.
- Hypertension.
- Osteoporosis.
- Increased blood sugar and protein metabolism.

Sonography
- Bilateral adrenal enlargement.
- Small nodules.

ADRENAL METASTASES

Lab/Symptoms
- Incidental finding.
- Adrenal hormones may be elevated.

Sonography
- Variable size.
- Usually bilateral.
- Solid well-defined lesion.

- Central necrosis may occur in larger lesions.
- May be difficult to separate from adenoma.

NEUROBLASTOMA

Lab/Symptoms

- Second most common mass in young children (Wilms' tumor is first).
- Asymptomatic.
- May present with anemia, failure to thrive, fever, increased catecholamines.

Sonography

- Heterogeneous mass with irregular borders.
- Calcifications common.
- Displaces kidney (Wilms' tumor compresses kidney).
- Look for associated nodes in paraaortic region and liver.

PHEOCHROMOCYTOMA

Lab/Symptoms

- May be asymptomatic or hypertensive.

Sonography

- Moderate size lesion (2 to 6 cm).
- Hypoechoic solid mass.
- Well encapsulated.
- Look for displacement of surrounding structures.

ABSCESSES AND POCKETS IN THE ABDOMEN AND PELVIS

ABSCESS: A cavity formed by necrosis within solid tissue or a circumscribed collection of purulent material. Abscesses will collect in the most dependent area of the body, thus all the "gutters" should be evaluated, the "pockets" and "pouches," and the spaces above and around various organs.

Lab/Symptoms
- Fever
- Chills
- Weakness
- Malaise
- Pain at the localized site of infection
- Liver function values normal
- Increased white blood cell
- Generalized sepsis
- Bacterial cultures (if superficial)

If an abscess is suspected (i.e., fever of unknown origin), the sonographer should evaluate these areas:
- Subdiaphragmatic (liver and spleen)
- Splenic recess and borders
- Hepatic recess and borders
- Liver/right kidney
- Pericolic gutters
- Lesser omentum
- Transverse mesocolon
- Morrison's pouch

- Gastrocolic ligament
- Phrenicosplenic ligament
- Recesses between intestinal loops and colon
- Extrahepatic falciform ligament
- Pouch of Douglas
- Broad ligaments (female)
- Anterior to urinary kidney

Sonography (General Appearance)

- Collections can appear quite varied in their texture due to length of time the abscess has formed, or the available space the abscess has to localize.
- Many collections may appear predominantly fluid-filled with irregular borders; they can also be complex with debris floating within the cystic mass, or they may be more of a solid pattern.
- If collection is in pelvis, careful analysis of bowel patterns and peristalsis should be made in attempts to separate the bowel from the abscess collection.
- Classically, an abscess appears as an elliptical sonolucent mass with thick and irregular margins.
- Abscesses tend to be under tension and tend to displace surrounding structures.
- Septated appearance may result from previous or developing adhesions.
- Necrotic debris produces low level internal echoes which may be seen to "float" within the abscess.
- Fluid levels are secondary to layering, probably because of the setting of debris.

Sonography of Gas-containing Abscess

- Present with varying echo patterns.
- Generally appear as a densely echogenic mass with or without acoustic shadowing and otherwise increased through transmission.

- A teratoma may mimic the pattern of a gas containing abscess, but the clinical history and x-ray will exclude them from the diagnosis.
- This type of abscess may be confused with a solid lesion because it may be difficult to determine the presence of through transmission.

Sonography of Peritonitis and Resultant Abscess Formation

- May be a generalized or localized process.
- Multiloculated abscesses or multiple collections should be documented and their size determined as accurately as possible to aid in planning drainage and for improved accuracy in follow-up studies.

Sonography of Lesser-sac Abscess

- Small "slit-like" epiploic foramen usually seals off the lesser sac from inflammatory processes extrinsic to it.
- If process begins within the lesser sac, such as with a pancreatic abscess, the sac may be involved in addition to other secondarily affected peritoneal and retroperitoneal spaces.
- Differential should include pseudocyst, pancreatic abscess, gastric outlet obstruction, fluid-filled stomach.

Sonography of Subphrenic Abscess

- LUQ difficult to examine.
- May alter patient's position to right lateral decubitus to scan along coronal plane of body or prone to use spleen as a window.
- Be careful of pleural effusions.
- May scan patient upright so pleural area and subdiaphragmatic area may be better demonstrated.

Sonography of Subcapsular Collections

- Fluid within liver may mimic loculated subphrenic fluid.
- Intraabdominal fluid may be differentiated by its smooth border and its tendency to conform to the contour of the liver; it displaces the

liver medially, rather than to indent the border locally, as subcapsular fluid might.
- A tense subphrenic abscess can displace the liver.
- May be difficult to distinguish subphrenic abscess from ascites.
- Can look at margins of the fluid collection to differentiate; or can look for other collections of fluid (in pelvis) to distinguish ascites from fluid.
- Preperitoneal fat anterior to the liver may mimic a localized fluid collection.

LIVER

Causes

Bacteria can enter the liver through five major pathways and cause abscess formation:
1. Through the portal system.
2. By way of ascending cholangitis of the common bile duct (most common cause in the United States).
3. Via the H.A. secondary to bacteremia.
4. By direct extension from an infection.
5. By implantation of bacteria after trauma to the abdominal wall.

RENAL

Renal abscesses are classified according to their locations.

Renal Carbuncle

An abscess that forms within the renal parenchyma.

Lab/Symptoms

- Varies from none to fever, leukocytosis, and flank pain.

Sonography

- Discrete mass within the kidney.
- May be cystic or cystic with debris or may be solid.

Perinephric Abscess

Usually the result of a perforated renal abscess that leaks purulent material into the tissues adjacent to the kidney.

Sonography

- Fluid collection around the kidney or an adjacent mass that can vary from a cystic to more solid appearance.

ABDOMINAL ABSCESS

Causes

- Surgery or trauma accounts for 85% of abdominal pelvic abscesses.

Notes

- Hepatic recesses and perihepatic spaces are most common sites for abscess.
- Pelvic region is a common site also (free fluid below the transverse mesocolon often flows into the pouch of Douglas and perivesical spaces).
- Right subhepatic space (fluid ascends up right pericolic gutter into Morrison's pouch, when fluid fills Morrison's pouch it spreads past the coronary ligament and up over the dome of the liver.
- Presence of a right subhepatic abscess generally implies previous contamination of the right subhepatic space.

APPENDICEAL ABSCESS

Acute appendicitis is the most common abdominal pathologic process that requires immediate surgery.

Cause

- Obstruction of the appendix is caused by a fecolith at its origin at the cecum.
- Appendix becomes distended rapidly after obstruction.

Symptoms
- Fever
- Severe pain near McBurney's point in RLQ (draw straight line between the umbilicus and the anterior superior iliac spine and then move 2 inches along the line from the iliac spine.

Lab
- Increased white blood cell

Differential Diagnosis
- Pelvic inflammatory disease.
- Twisted or ruptured ovarian cyst.
- Acute gastroenteritis.
- Mesenteric lymphadenitis.

Sonography
- Complex RLQ mass.
- Examine other gutters to R/O differentials.

ABDOMINAL WALL MASSES
Usually occur after surgery.

Sonography
- May have cystic, complex, or solid characteristics.
- Generally are very superficial, easy to locate and tap if necessary.

HEMATOMA

Causes
- Surgical injury to tissue and blunt or sharp trauma to the abdomen.

Lab
- Lab values may show decrease in hematocrit and red blood cells.
- Patient may go into shock.

Sonography

- Depends on the stage of the bleed.
- New bleeds are primarily cystic with some debris (blood clots); as the blood begins to organize, the mass becomes more "solid" in appearance.
- New clots may be very homogeneous.
- Hematomas may become infected and at any stage may be sonographically indistinguishable from abscess; they may mimic subphrenic fluid.

LYMPHOCELES

Notes

- Collections generally look like loculated, simple fluid collections, although they may have a more complex, usually separated morphology.
- Differentiation from loculated ascites is usually possible because the mass effect of a lymphocele that is under tension will displace the surrounding organs.
- Differentiation from other fluid collections is mainly made by aspiration.

PERITONEUM

Notes

- Peritoneal lining is not seen as a distinct structure during sonography unless it is thickened.
- Is usually secondary to metastatic implants or to direct extension of tumor from the viscera or mesentery.
- Primary mesotheliomas occur rarely.